Food Experiment

30 Days to Finding What You Love to Eat!

Jessica Wallaker

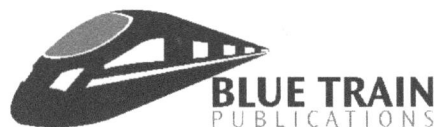

BLUE TRAIN
PUBLICATIONS

Published by Blue Train Publications in 2017

First Edition; First Printing

© 2017 Jessica Wallaker

Rcksldgym.com

Cover background image from Engin_Akyurt

ISBN **978-0-9996436-0-0**

Dedication

I dedicate this book to you! As you go through this, my hope is that you enjoy the experience and aren't too hard on yourself. Finding YOUR food and what works best for you is an amazing and freeing experience. I hope you have as much fun with it as I did.

Here we go!

What to do

- This is supposed to be fun! So make sure you come into this with an open mind and pure curiosity. No regrets, negative thinking; this is just an experiment. So here's how it works!

- Use each day and finish through for 30 days. Even if you skip a day or 2, just practice keeping track of how you're feeling and any other areas you can fill out.

- Start with putting down how much sleep you got, then circle either "Rested" or "Tired". This will help you find out what's working during the day and then also how much sleep YOU need.

- You will be filling out this journal throughout the day. So if stressors start to come up, write them down. This way they are out of your head and will seem more manageable to deal with.

- Now, this is NOT a diet journal. This is a food journal. So write down your meals, what all you had and don't worry about calories. If the meal came from a recipe you tried, write down where you got it so you can find it again.

- Next if you end up snacking, write down what you had and at what time. This will help you have an idea what meals keep you fuller longer and what meals don't satisfy you enough. Do this through breakfast and dinner, be honest and curious what happens.

- Once you have made it through the day, answer the questions at the end: "How did you feel throughout the day?", "Did you have enough energy?", "What's one meal you really enjoyed and why?", and "Did you stress eat?"

- At the end of the week, go back and review. Write down your thoughts of the week, good and bad so you know moving forward what's going on. Be honest, this is for you!

- All of these questions are to help you find what works best for you and if you are using food to cope throughout the day. Use this as an experiment for what works and what doesn't, what you like and don't like, and how it has an affect on your day.

- The only way you can fail is by not eating. So stick with it, have fun, treat yourself, and see what happens after 30 days of eating!

Enjoy!

Perfection is not attainable, but if we chase perfection we can catch excellence.

Vince Lombardi

What I would love to see happen in the next 30 days and why

_____
_____
_____
_____
_____
_____
_____
_____
_____
_____
_____
_____
_____
_____
_____
_____
_____

___/ ___/ ____

Sleep:___ **Rested** or **Tired**

Stressors of the Day:

1. _____

2. _____

3. _____

Breakfast

Recipe:

Snacks?

What time?

Lunch

Recipe:

Snacks?

What time?

Dinner

Recipe:

Snacks?

What time?

How did you feel throughout the day?

_____

_____

_____

_____

_____

Did you have enough energy?

_____

_____

_____

_____

What's one meal you really enjoyed and why?

_____

_____

_____

_____

Did you stress eat?

_____

_____

_____

___/ ___/ ____

Sleep:___ **Rested** or **Tired**

Stressors of the Day:

1. _____

2. _____

3. _____

Breakfast	Lunch
Recipe:	Recipe:
Snacks? What time?	Snacks? What time?

Dinner

Recipe:

Snacks?

What time?

How did you feel throughout the day?

_____

_____

_____

_____

_____

Did you have enough energy?

_____

_____

_____

_____

What's one meal you really enjoyed and why?

_____

_____

_____

_____

Did you stress eat?

_____

_____

_____

___ / ___ / ____

Sleep:___ **Rested** or **Tired**

Stressors of the Day:

1. _____

2. _____

3. _____

Breakfast

Recipe:

Snacks?

What time?

Lunch

Recipe:

Snacks?

What time?

Dinner

Recipe:

Snacks?

What time?

Day Review:

How did you feel throughout the day?

_____

_____

_____

_____

_____

Did you have enough energy?

_____

_____

_____

_____

What's one meal you really enjoyed and why?

_____

_____

_____

_____

Did you stress eat?

_____

_____

_____

___/ ___/ ____

Sleep:___ **Rested** or **Tired**

Stressors of the Day:

1. _____

2. _____

3. _____

Breakfast

Recipe:

Snacks?

What time?

Lunch

Recipe:

Snacks?

What time?

Dinner

Recipe:

Snacks?

What time?

How did you feel throughout the day?

_____
_____
_____
_____
_____

Did you have enough energy?

_____
_____
_____
_____

What's one meal you really enjoyed and why?

_____
_____
_____
_____

Did you stress eat?

_____
_____
_____

___/ ___/ ____

Sleep:___ **Rested** or **Tired**

Stressors of the Day:

1. _____

2. _____

3. _____

Breakfast	Lunch
Recipe:	Recipe:
Snacks?	Snacks?
What time?	What time?

Dinner

Recipe:

Snacks?

What time?

How did you feel throughout the day?

_____

_____

_____

_____

_____

Did you have enough energy?

_____

_____

_____

_____

What's one meal you really enjoyed and why?

_____

_____

_____

_____

Did you stress eat?

_____

_____

_____

___/ ___/ ____

Sleep:___ **Rested** or **Tired**

Stressors of the Day:

1. _____

2. _____

3. _____

Breakfast	Lunch
Recipe:	Recipe:
Snacks?	Snacks?
What time?	What time?

Dinner

Recipe:

Snacks?

What time?

How did you feel throughout the day?

_____
_____
_____
_____
_____

Did you have enough energy?

_____
_____
_____
_____

What's one meal you really enjoyed and why?

_____
_____
_____

Did you stress eat?

_____
_____
_____

___/ ___/ ____

Sleep:___ **Rested** or **Tired**

Stressors of the Day:

1. _____

2. _____

3. _____

Breakfast	Lunch
Recipe:	Recipe:
Snacks?	Snacks?
What time?	What time?

Dinner

Recipe:

Snacks?

What time?

Day Review:

How did you feel throughout the day?

_____

_____

_____

_____

_____

Did you have enough energy?

_____

_____

_____

_____

What's one meal you really enjoyed and why?

_____

_____

_____

_____

Did you stress eat?

_____

_____

_____

Week Overview

What did you find out this week?

_____

_____

_____

_____

_____

Were you surprised by anything that came up? Food issues, snacking, cravings, feelings, etc?

_____

_____

_____

_____

_____

Any foods/recipes you enjoyed and want to try again? **Y** or **N**

If yes, what were they??

Further Thoughts

Upcoming Days Events

Any stressors you need to prep for these coming days?

- _____
  _____

- _____
  _____

- _____
  _____

- _____
  _____

- _____
  _____

- _____
  _____

- _____
  _____

Your diet is a bank account. Good food choices are good investments.
Bethenny Frankel

Final thoughts heading into the next round:

_____

_____

_____

_____

_____

_____

_____

_____

_____

_____

_____

_____

_____

___/ ___/ ____

Sleep:___ **Rested** or **Tired**

Stressors of the Day:

1. _____

2. _____

3. _____

Breakfast	Lunch
Recipe:	Recipe:
Snacks? What time?	Snacks? What time?

Dinner

Recipe:

Snacks?

What time?

Day Review:

How did you feel throughout the day?

_____
_____
_____
_____
_____

Did you have enough energy?

_____
_____
_____
_____

What's one meal you really enjoyed and why?

_____
_____
_____
_____

Did you stress eat?

_____
_____
_____

___/___/____

Sleep:___ **Rested** or **Tired**

Stressors of the Day:

1. _____

2. _____

3. _____

Breakfast

Recipe:

Snacks?

What time?

Lunch

Recipe:

Snacks?

What time?

Dinner

Recipe:

Snacks?

What time?

How did you feel throughout the day?

_____

_____

_____

_____

_____

Did you have enough energy?

_____

_____

_____

_____

What's one meal you really enjoyed and why?

_____

_____

_____

_____

Did you stress eat?

_____

_____

_____

___/ ___/ ____

Sleep:___ **Rested** or **Tired**

Stressors of the Day:

1. _____

2. _____

3. _____

Breakfast	Lunch
Recipe:	Recipe:
Snacks? What time?	Snacks? What time?

Dinner

Recipe:

Snacks?

What time?

How did you feel throughout the day?

_____

_____

_____

_____

_____

Did you have enough energy?

_____

_____

_____

_____

What's one meal you really enjoyed and why?

_____

_____

_____

_____

Did you stress eat?

_____

_____

_____

___/___/____

Sleep:___ **Rested** or **Tired**

Stressors of the Day:

1. _____

2. _____

3. _____

Breakfast

Recipe:

Snacks?

What time?

Lunch

Recipe:

Snacks?

What time?

Dinner

Recipe:

Snacks?

What time?

How did you feel throughout the day?

_____

_____

_____

_____

_____

Did you have enough energy?

_____

_____

_____

_____

What's one meal you really enjoyed and why?

_____

_____

_____

_____

Did you stress eat?

_____

_____

_____

___/ ___/ ____

Sleep:___ **Rested** or **Tired**

Stressors of the Day:

1. _____

2. _____

3. _____

Breakfast	Lunch
Recipe:	Recipe:
Snacks?	Snacks?
What time?	What time?

Dinner

Recipe:

Snacks?

What time?

How did you feel throughout the day?

_____

_____

_____

_____

_____

Did you have enough energy?

_____

_____

_____

_____

What's one meal you really enjoyed and why?

_____

_____

_____

Did you stress eat?

_____

_____

_____

___/ ___/ _____

Sleep:___ **Rested** or **Tired**

Stressors of the Day:

1. _____

2. _____

3. _____

Breakfast	Lunch
Recipe:	Recipe:
Snacks?	Snacks?
What time?	What time?

Dinner

Recipe:

Snacks?

What time?

How did you feel throughout the day?

_____

_____

_____

_____

_____

Did you have enough energy?

_____

_____

_____

_____

What's one meal you really enjoyed and why?

_____

_____

_____

_____

Did you stress eat?

_____

_____

_____

___/___/___

Sleep:___ **Rested** or **Tired**

Stressors of the Day:

1. _____

2. _____

3. _____

Breakfast

Recipe:

Snacks?

What time?

Lunch

Recipe:

Snacks?

What time?

Dinner

Recipe:

Snacks?

What time?

How did you feel throughout the day?

_____
_____
_____
_____
_____

Did you have enough energy?

_____
_____
_____
_____

What's one meal you really enjoyed and why?

_____
_____
_____

Did you stress eat?

_____
_____
_____

Week Overview

What did you find out this week?

_____

_____

_____

_____

_____

Were you surprised by anything that came up? Food issues, snacking, cravings, feelings, etc?

_____

_____

_____

_____

_____

Any foods/recipes you enjoyed and want to try again? **Y** or **N**

If yes, what were they??

Further Thoughts

Upcoming Days Events

Any stressors you need to prep for these coming days?

- _____
  _____

- _____
  _____

- _____
  _____

- _____
  _____

- _____
  _____

- _____
  _____

- _____
  _____

Good food is healthy food. Food is supposed to sustain you so you can live better, not so you can eat more. Some people eat to live, and some people live to eat.

Yolanda Adams

Final thoughts heading into the next round:

_____

_____

_____

_____

_____

_____

_____

_____

_____

_____

_____

_____

_____

___/___/____

Sleep:___ **Rested** or **Tired**

Stressors of the Day:

1. _____

2. _____

3. _____

Breakfast	Lunch
Recipe:	Recipe:
Snacks?	Snacks?
What time?	What time?

Dinner

Recipe:

Snacks?

What time?

Day Review:

How did you feel throughout the day?

_____

_____

_____

_____

_____

Did you have enough energy?

_____

_____

_____

_____

What's one meal you really enjoyed and why?

_____

_____

_____

_____

Did you stress eat?

_____

_____

_____

___/ ___/ ____

Sleep:___ **Rested** or **Tired**

Stressors of the Day:

1. _____

2. _____

3. _____

Breakfast

Recipe:

Snacks?

What time?

Lunch

Recipe:

Snacks?

What time?

Dinner

Recipe:

Snacks?

What time?

How did you feel throughout the day?

_____

_____

_____

_____

_____

Did you have enough energy?

_____

_____

_____

_____

What's one meal you really enjoyed and why?

_____

_____

_____

Did you stress eat?

_____

_____

_____

___/ ___/ ____

Sleep:___ **Rested** or **Tired**

Stressors of the Day:

1. _____

2. _____

3. _____

Breakfast	Lunch
Recipe:	Recipe:
Snacks?	Snacks?
What time?	What time?

Dinner

Recipe:

Snacks?

What time?

How did you feel throughout the day?

_____

_____

_____

_____

_____

Did you have enough energy?

_____

_____

_____

_____

What's one meal you really enjoyed and why?

_____

_____

_____

_____

Did you stress eat?

_____

_____

_____

___/___/___

Sleep:___ **Rested** or **Tired**

Stressors of the Day:

1. _____

2. _____

3. _____

Breakfast

Recipe:

Snacks?

What time?

Lunch

Recipe:

Snacks?

What time?

Dinner

Recipe:

Snacks?

What time?

Day Review:

How did you feel throughout the day?

_____

_____

_____

_____

_____

Did you have enough energy?

_____

_____

_____

_____

What's one meal you really enjoyed and why?

_____

_____

_____

_____

Did you stress eat?

_____

_____

_____

___/ ___/ ____

Sleep:___ **Rested** or **Tired**

Stressors of the Day:

1. _____

2. _____

3. _____

Breakfast

Recipe:

Snacks?

What time?

Lunch

Recipe:

Snacks?

What time?

Dinner

Recipe:

Snacks?

What time?

Day Review:

How did you feel throughout the day?

_____

_____

_____

_____

_____

Did you have enough energy?

_____

_____

_____

_____

What's one meal you really enjoyed and why?

_____

_____

_____

_____

Did you stress eat?

_____

_____

_____

___/ ___/ ____

Sleep:___ **Rested** or **Tired**

Stressors of the Day:

1. _____

2. _____

3. _____

Breakfast

Recipe:

Snacks?

What time?

Lunch

Recipe:

Snacks?

What time?

Day Review:

Dinner

Recipe:

Snacks?

What time?

How did you feel throughout the day?

_____

_____

_____

_____

_____

Did you have enough energy?

_____

_____

_____

_____

What's one meal you really enjoyed and why?

_____

_____

_____

Did you stress eat?

_____

_____

_____

___/___/____

Sleep:___ **Rested** or **Tired**

Stressors of the Day:

1. _____

2. _____

3. _____

Breakfast

Recipe:

Snacks?

What time?

Lunch

Recipe:

Snacks?

What time?

Dinner

Recipe:

Snacks?

What time?

How did you feel throughout the day?

_____
_____
_____
_____
_____

Did you have enough energy?

_____
_____
_____
_____

What's one meal you really enjoyed and why?

_____
_____
_____
_____

Did you stress eat?

_____
_____
_____

Week Overview

What did you find out this week?

_____

_____

_____

_____

_____

Were you surprised by anything that came up? Food issues, snacking, cravings, feelings, etc?

_____

_____

_____

_____

_____

Any foods/recipes you enjoyed and want to try again? **Y** or **N**

If yes, what were they??

Further Thoughts

Upcoming Days Events

Any stressors you need to prep for these coming days?

- _____
  _____
- _____
  _____
- _____
  _____
- _____
  _____
- _____
  _____
- _____
  _____

When you rise in the morning, give thanks for the light, for your life, for your strength. Give thanks for your food and for the joy of living. If you see no reason to give thanks, the fault lies in yourself.

Tecumseh

Final thoughts heading into the next round:

_____

_____

_____

_____

_____

_____

_____

_____

_____

_____

_____

_____

_____

___/ ___/ ____

Sleep:___ **Rested** or **Tired**

Stressors of the Day:

1. _____

2. _____

3. _____

Breakfast

Recipe:

Snacks?

What time?

Lunch

Recipe:

Snacks?

What time?

Dinner

Recipe:

Snacks?

What time?

Day Review:

How did you feel throughout the day?

_____

_____

_____

_____

_____

Did you have enough energy?

_____

_____

_____

_____

What's one meal you really enjoyed and why?

_____

_____

_____

Did you stress eat?

_____

_____

_____

___/___/___

Sleep:___ **Rested** or **Tired**

Stressors of the Day:

1. _____

2. _____

3. _____

Breakfast

Recipe:

Snacks?

What time?

Lunch

Recipe:

Snacks?

What time?

Dinner

Recipe:

Snacks?

What time?

How did you feel throughout the day?

_____

_____

_____

_____

_____

Did you have enough energy?

_____

_____

_____

_____

What's one meal you really enjoyed and why?

_____

_____

_____

_____

Did you stress eat?

_____

_____

_____

___/ ___/ ____

Sleep:___ **Rested** or **Tired**

Stressors of the Day:

1. _____

2. _____

3. _____

Breakfast	Lunch
Recipe:	Recipe:
Snacks?	Snacks?
What time?	What time?

Dinner

Recipe:

Snacks?

What time?

How did you feel throughout the day?

_____

_____

_____

_____

_____

Did you have enough energy?

_____

_____

_____

_____

What's one meal you really enjoyed and why?

_____

_____

_____

_____

Did you stress eat?

_____

_____

_____

___/___/___

Sleep:___ **Rested** or **Tired**

Stressors of the Day:

1. _____

2. _____

3. _____

Breakfast

Recipe:

Snacks?

What time?

Lunch

Recipe:

Snacks?

What time?

Dinner

Recipe:

Snacks?

What time?

How did you feel throughout the day?

_____

_____

_____

_____

_____

Did you have enough energy?

_____

_____

_____

_____

What's one meal you really enjoyed and why?

_____

_____

_____

_____

Did you stress eat?

_____

_____

_____

___/ ___/ ____

Stressors of the Day:

1. _____

2. _____

3. _____

Sleep:___ **Rested** or **Tired**

Breakfast

Recipe:

Snacks?

What time?

Lunch

Recipe:

Snacks?

What time?

Dinner

Recipe:

Snacks?

What time?

How did you feel throughout the day?

_____

_____

_____

_____

_____

Did you have enough energy?

_____

_____

_____

_____

What's one meal you really enjoyed and why?

_____

_____

_____

_____

Did you stress eat?

_____

_____

_____

___/___/___

Sleep:___ **Rested** or **Tired**

Stressors of the Day:

1. _____

2. _____

3. _____

Breakfast

Recipe:

Snacks?

What time?

Lunch

Recipe:

Snacks?

What time?

Dinner

Recipe:

Snacks?

What time?

How did you feel throughout the day?

_____

_____

_____

_____

_____

Did you have enough energy?

_____

_____

_____

_____

What's one meal you really enjoyed and why?

_____

_____

_____

_____

Did you stress eat?

_____

_____

_____

___/___/____

Sleep:___ **Rested** or **Tired**

Stressors of the Day:

1. _____

2. _____

3. _____

Breakfast	Lunch
Recipe:	Recipe:
Snacks?	Snacks?
What time?	What time?

Dinner

Recipe:

Snacks?

What time?

How did you feel throughout the day?

_____

_____

_____

_____

_____

Did you have enough energy?

_____

_____

_____

_____

What's one meal you really enjoyed and why?

_____

_____

_____

_____

Did you stress eat?

_____

_____

_____

Week Overview

What did you find out this week?

_____

_____

_____

_____

_____

Were you surprised by anything that came up? Food issues, snacking, cravings, feelings, etc?

_____

_____

_____

_____

_____

Any foods/recipes you enjoyed and want to try again? **Y** or **N**

If yes, what were they??

Further Thoughts

Upcoming Days Events

Any stressors you need to prep for these coming days?

- _____
  _____

- _____
  _____

- _____
  _____

- _____
  _____

- _____
  _____

- _____
  _____

- _____
  _____

Let food be thy medicine and medicine be thy food.

Hippocrates

Final thoughts heading into the next round:

_____

_____

_____

_____

_____

_____

_____

_____

_____

_____

_____

_____

_____

_____

___/___/____

Sleep:___ **Rested** or **Tired**

Stressors of the Day:

1. _____

2. _____

3. _____

Breakfast

Recipe:

Snacks?

What time?

Lunch

Recipe:

Snacks?

What time?

Dinner

Recipe:

Snacks?

What time?

How did you feel throughout the day?

_____

_____

_____

_____

_____

Did you have enough energy?

_____

_____

_____

_____

What's one meal you really enjoyed and why?

_____

_____

_____

_____

Did you stress eat?

_____

_____

_____

___/___/____

Sleep:___ **Rested** or **Tired**

Stressors of the Day:

1. _____

2. _____

3. _____

Breakfast	Lunch
Recipe:	Recipe:
Snacks?	Snacks?
What time?	What time?

Dinner

Recipe:

Snacks?

What time?

Day Review:

How did you feel throughout the day?

_____

_____

_____

_____

_____

Did you have enough energy?

_____

_____

_____

_____

What's one meal you really enjoyed and why?

_____

_____

_____

Did you stress eat?

_____

_____

_____

30 Days!

You made it to the end of your 30 days! What have you found out about yourself?

_____

_____

_____

_____

_____

Were you surprised by the foods/meals your body enjoys?

_____

_____

_____

_____

_____

Was this beneficial for you? **Y** or **N**

Overall Thoughts

_____

_____

_____

_____

_____

_____

_____

_____

_____

_____

_____

_____

_____

_____

_____

_____

_____

_____

Next Step

There will be spots to finish out the week, so do that and then come back. Bonus!

NOW:

Is this something you feel you can keep going with?

_____
_____
_____
_____

Are you happy and comfortable with how this fits in with your life?

_____
_____
_____
_____
_____

Is there anything that will make it hard for you to keep making progress?

_____

_____

_____

_____

_____

What will be beneficial for you to have in order to keep going forward with your goals?

_____

_____

_____

_____

_____

I have faith in you! If you've truly filled out this journal and made it to the end, however that looks for you, you finished something! And that's a great thing in itself! Don't let the fact that this is done stop you from progressing on. Do what you must to stay motivated. You've got this. Now, on to the next experiment!

~ Jessie

___/___/___

Sleep:___ **Rested** or **Tired**

Stressors of the Day:

1. _____

2. _____

3. _____

Breakfast

Recipe:

Snacks?

What time?

Lunch

Recipe:

Snacks?

What time?

Dinner

Recipe:

Snacks?

What time?

How did you feel throughout the day?

_____

_____

_____

_____

_____

Did you have enough energy?

_____

_____

_____

_____

What's one meal you really enjoyed and why?

_____

_____

_____

_____

Did you stress eat?

_____

_____

_____

___/___/____

Sleep:___ **Rested** or **Tired**

Stressors of the Day:

1. _____

2. _____

3. _____

Breakfast

Recipe:

Snacks?

What time?

Lunch

Recipe:

Snacks?

What time?

Dinner

Recipe:

Snacks?

What time?

How did you feel throughout the day?

_____

_____

_____

_____

_____

Did you have enough energy?

_____

_____

_____

_____

What's one meal you really enjoyed and why?

_____

_____

_____

Did you stress eat?

_____

_____

_____

___/ ___/ ____

Sleep:___ **Rested** or **Tired**

Stressors of the Day:

1. _____

2. _____

3. _____

Breakfast

Recipe:

Snacks?

What time?

Lunch

Recipe:

Snacks?

What time?

Dinner

Recipe:

Snacks?

What time?

How did you feel throughout the day?

_____

_____

_____

_____

_____

Did you have enough energy?

_____

_____

_____

_____

What's one meal you really enjoyed and why?

_____

_____

_____

Did you stress eat?

_____

_____

_____

___/ ___/ ____

Sleep:___ **Rested** or **Tired**

Stressors of the Day:

1. _____

2. _____

3. _____

Breakfast

Recipe:

Snacks?

What time?

Lunch

Recipe:

Snacks?

What time?

Dinner

Recipe:

Snacks?

What time?

How did you feel throughout the day?

_____
_____
_____
_____
_____

Did you have enough energy?

_____
_____
_____
_____

What's one meal you really enjoyed and why?

_____
_____
_____

Did you stress eat?

_____
_____
_____

___/___/_____

Sleep:___ **Rested** or **Tired**

Stressors of the Day:

1. _____

2. _____

3. _____

Breakfast

Recipe:

Snacks?

What time?

Lunch

Recipe:

Snacks?

What time?

Dinner

Recipe:

Snacks?

What time?

How did you feel throughout the day?

_____

_____

_____

_____

_____

Did you have enough energy?

_____

_____

_____

_____

What's one meal you really enjoyed and why?

_____

_____

_____

Did you stress eat?

_____

_____

_____

Don't judge each day by the harvest you reap but by the seeds that you plant.

Robert Louis Stevenson

What I would love to see happen in the next 30 days and why

_____
_____
_____
_____
_____
_____
_____
_____
_____
_____
_____
_____
_____
_____
_____
_____
_____
_____
_____

About the Author

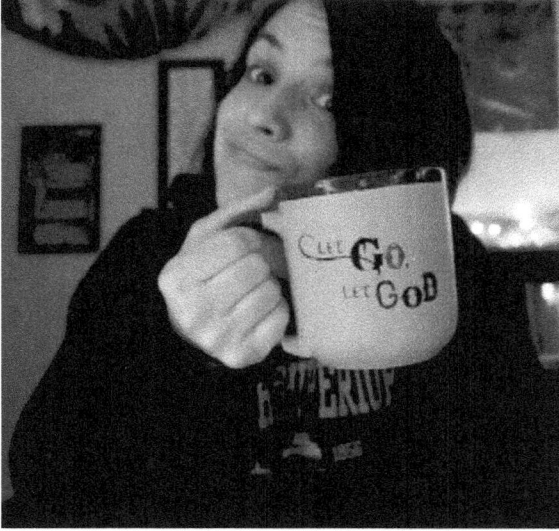

Confident and Fit Coaching
rcksldgym.com

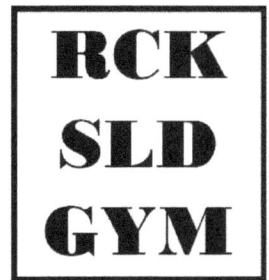

RCK
SLD
GYM

Jessica Wallaker is a young entrepreneur in the making. From starting her own coaching business, Confident and Fit Coaching, in her early 20's to writing her first journal in 2017. Her main goal with coaching and writing is to help people better understand what it is that they want to get out of their life. Showing them that health doesn't have to be one separate compartment in their hectic schedule; it can be fun, enjoyable and also stress free. Who would've thought!

If you are interested in any coaching or upcoming programs, please go to rcksldgym.com

So be sure to follow her on social media or check out her website to keep up-to-date on all the new adventures and endeavors she is trying out today.

Also By Jessica Wallaker

Movement Experiment

30 Days to Finding How You Love to Move!

Jessica Wallaker

Available at amazon.com
Be sure to check us out at rcksldgym.com for new additions coming soon!